High Energy Herbs

Powerful Herbs for Energy and Longevity

Richard Anderson

To all those who choose a different
way

Disclaimer

The information provided in this book is designed to provide useful information on the subjects discussed. This book is not meant to be used, nor should it be used, to diagnose or treat any medical condition. For diagnosis or treatment of a medical problem, consult your own physician. The publisher and author are not responsible for any health or allergy needs that may require medical supervision and are not liable for any damages or negative consequences from any treatment, action, application or preparation, to any person reading or following the information in this book. References are provided for informational purposes only and do not constitute endorsement of any website or other sources. Readers should be aware that the websites listed in this book may change.

Table of Contents

Introduction

This is a book about herbs and the powerful effect they can have on our energy, vitality and longevity. It is very likely you already know that herbs can dramatically affect our bodies and health or you wouldn't be reading this book. Some powerful Herbs can be wonderful additions to our daily routines and can have amazingly wonderful effects on our energy, our appearance and our vitality. This book will give you a great introduction to several powerful herbs and explain how to use them in your daily life.

I've always been attracted to herbs and started using them when I was a teenager. It was so exciting to see amazing results from the herbs in a very short period of time. Although I was just a teenager, I was always brewing new concoctions and trying new herbs. As I got older I regularly used herbs to enhance my daily. I even found that I could use herbs to enhance my senses when I began running and increase my overall joy of physical activity.

As the years went by I would share some of my most dramatic herbal discoveries with a few people if I felt they were open to it.

Some of the results were really life changing when they used the herbs properly and gave the plants a chance to do their magic. Much of the feedback came in the form of 'you should write a book', so here is my energy herb book. It's a book about some of my favorite and most life enhancing herbs for energy, vitality and longevity.

I've included a few valuable terms used in traditional Chinese medicine. Its valuable to at least have a slight familiarity with the terms as you continue on with your herbal adventures. I've really tried to explain the terms in a very simplified way so everyone could grasp their meaning right away.

Some of the 'herbs' in this book aren't considered herbs by many, but I've included them anyway because they are important plant based substances that have a wonderful effect on your energy levels.

You'll also find a fairly thorough question and answer section so you won't feel lost along the way.

Be sure to give the herbs a chance and form a long term relationship with them. It's not an accident that the herbs are so compatible with us. Nature gave these to us to heal, enhance and restore our bodies. They really are magical and wonderful gifts from the earth to us. Accept the gift!

Richard Anderson February 2014

Chapter 1 Herbs for Energy Vitality and Longevity

In this section I outline and discuss several herbs that are known to have an energizing effect on the skin and body. They increase circulation of life force and raise the vitality level of the body. They don't just increase your energy; surprisingly, they often enhance your appearance as well. True beauty isn't really perfectly balanced features, it's the level of vitality and/or strength of life force a person exudes throughout their system. These herbs really have multiple positive effects on your physicality. I chose these herbs because I have used them often and seen dramatic results. These herbs will not only help you to appear healthier and increase your energy but many are also longevity extending herbs that tend to increase the lifespan of people using them for long periods of time. However, there are so many energy and life-enhancing herbs out there that I couldn't cover them all in this book, but will likely include more of them in a companion book.

American Ginseng:

American Ginseng is a great energizing herb that is also very cooling. Massive amounts of American Ginseng are consumed by the Chinese, especially in the summer to deal with the brutal heat and humidity of China. If you walk through a local Chinatown in the States you see often see giant drums of American Ginseng in the front of the stores because it is such a big seller. Surprising fact, most of it is grown in Wisconsin and shipped to China. As with many of the root herbs bigger is often better and more costly. It makes sense because a bigger root stays in the ground longer and has a chance to develop more active constituents. Take heart though as even the younger, smaller and cheaper roots give a noticeable energizing effect within a few hours. **Dosage is one 500 mg capsules or one or 2 slices as tea in hot water or slowly chewed.**

Ashwagandha:

Ashwagandha is a powerful herb for the mind and body. It is a wonderful rejuvenating herb that balances and nourishes the entire system. Most people notice its energy enhancing effects within days, but its best effects occur after weeks of use. This herb is incredible as it does so many wonderful things in the body! To name a few; it help protects the kidneys, liver and heart, lifts the mood, helps you sleep better and is powerfully anti-inflammatory. Also your ability to handle stress will be greatly enhanced along with increases of physical and mental energy throughout the day. If you're like most who try it you will be glad that you added this wonderful herb to your regular regimen. **Dosage is two 500 mg capsules or one or two 250 mg extract.**

Cordyceps:
Cordyceps is a type of fungus that grows on the back of worms and is also now cultivated without the worms. It is an incredible energy and rejuvenation tonic that is great for the kidneys and liver. Until recently it was only available in Chinese herbs shops at very high prices which made it impractical to take by the average consumer. Now high quality cultivated Cordyceps is available in extract form at very reasonable prices. I have found it to be a very fast acting and outstanding herbal product to take. This is one of those herbs that a person will usually feel within days and sometimes within hours of trying it. **Dosage is two 500 mg capsules or one 250 mg extract.**

Cayenne:

Most people just see Cayenne as a spice that makes food hot but there is much more to this great herb. Cayenne is a very reliable and quick acting stimulant to the entire system. When you take cayenne you are definitely going to quickly notice its effects. It's very hot and energizing and like ginger, will enhance the effects of the other herbs in this book. You'll notice a pleasant warmth and energy spreading throughout your system in a very short period of time. People find that it can be a great hangover cure if used with lots of water. I like to have cayenne and ginger capsules handy when I travel or visit friends. I know that if I've gotten too cold they will always warm me from within and I can avoid catJing a cold. Always buy the deepest red cayenne you can find as I have found it is a sign of freshness. **Dosage is one or two 500 mg capsules.**

Cinnamon:

Cinnamon isn't just a delicious hot spice, it is very energizing and invigoration to the system. I love the smell and taste of fresh sweet cinnamon powder. It's so unique and wonderful. Unfortunately many people have never experienced this because the cinnamon powder they buy at a supermarket was ground months or even years before they bought it and most of the incredible volatile oils that make it so special have been lost with time. Always buy the freshest ground cinnamon you can find. I'm lucky enough to have a Costco close by that sells fresh powdered Cinnamon from Saigon. It's amazingly fresh and the price is fantastic! If Costco isn't an option for you try online sources of spices with companies that have a reputation for fresh spices and herbs. Swanson Vitamins is usually pretty reliable when it comes to the freshness of spices, so that could be another option for you. It has been getting a lot of notice lately because one of its abilities is to balance blood sugar levels in some people that suffer with high or low blood sugar. Balancing blood sugar is just one of its attributes. It is an amazing spice that is powerfully invigorating to your circulatory system and also has wonderful antibiotic qualities. One way of using it is to simply use it on it's own when you're feeling cold or you can mix it with other herbs like ginger and cayenne for an extra warming energy boost. As with all the warming herbs, monitor yourself as you use it. If you are feeling too warm after using it for awhile stop using it for a week or two and add Red Dates and Wolf berries to your daily schdule to cool and normalize the system. I don't recommend using the extract as I believe the extracting process removes many of the beneficial properties. **Dosage is 1 teaspoon or 2 500 mg capsules.**

Dendrobium Nobile:

Dendrobium, or Shi Hu in Chinese, is a variety of orchid cultivated for herbal applications. The stems and pods are both used, but most of the useful properties are concentrated in the pods. Dendrobium is a great restorative and longevity herb. It's a cooling, or Yin herb, that especially benefits the kidneys and eyes. It infuses powerful regenerative and restorative energy back into the body so it will be there when you need it. This herb is actually a beautiful golden color when it's good quality. It's almost like nature wanted us to pay attention to this herb. This is great to use if you've been working or playing too hard and feel really depleted. I like to go to Chinatown and pick some of the best golden pods and stems I can find but I know this isn't feasible for most people. In Chinatown you can also find it in the shape of a golden flattened sprig. The larger sizes are preferred but more expensive. Your best bet might be to buy concentrated powdered extracts online. A small bottle of powdered extract can be kind of pricey, but it lasts quite awhile so it's worth the money. Use up a bottle every other month for deep renewal, cooling and longevity. If you are lucky enough to have a Chinatown close by I recommend you buy it there but remember good quality Shi Hu (pronounced she hoo or sheh hoo) is costly. One of the reasons it's so expensive is that it takes along time to grow and cultivate. If you do end up going to Chinatown to buy it, take it by brewing approximately a level teaspoon in 3 cups of water on low heat (not boiling) in a covered glass pot for up to 3 hours. You can redo this process two more times. It has to be a slow heat extraction process because the herb is very dense and you don't want to boil it, because you can boil away its beneficial properties. **Dosage is one half teaspoon extract powder once or twice a day.**

Ginger:
Ahhh, Ginger! For most people, Ginger is great herb to take everyday. It's very stimulating and energizing. It's good to take with your other herbs as it enhances their circulation in your system. I believe it actually helps to open the acupuncture channels and meridians in the body so your life force can flow more freely throughout your system. The easiest way to take Ginger is in capsule form or you can buy raw ginger

from the supermarket. I like to slice off a piece of fresh Ginger and just chew it up and spit out the pulpish residue, but many people find this too intense. However, if you do buy fresh Ginger, keep it in the refrigerator or it will probably start to mold and spoil quickly.

Please don't take too much ginger! My friend loved all the amazing effects of Ginger and decided he was going to get even more benefits by drinking Ginger juice several times a day. Ginger is a very hot herb and very energizing and the juice almost completely unbalanced his body as he had severely over-heated his system. He called me, terrified, asking for help and I recommended some cooling herbs that balanced him out in 24 hours. Some herbs like Ginger are especially powerful and should never be abused. I don't recommend an extract of ginger because I think you're better off just using the fresh herb or fresh powder. **Dosage is one 1/8 inch slice, or one or two 500 mg powder capsules.**

Gokshura:
Gokshura, or Tribulus, is another herb that I use on a daily basis. It's not a stimulant

but an incredible power-increasing herb that you begin notice after taking it for a week or two. This is a tried and true herb that has been used in India for thousands of years! It strengthens and protects the kidneys and liver and helps to rejuvenate them over time. After taking this herb for awhile you will be stronger, more powerful and centered. It also increases the amount of available testosterone in men. The latest scientific research shows it also has great benefits in increasing blood circulation in the heart! This is one herb that I recommend only taking an extract because I found it seems to work in a more reliable way. All the extracts that I have tested seem to be of good quality. **Dosage is one or two 500 mg extract capsules.**

Green Tea:
Green tea is a wonderful way to increase ones energy throughout the day. This is one of my preferred energizers. It's very tasty and easy to use. Green tea contains so many health enhancing powers that if I listed them all it would just be ridiculous. So I will list just a few of the most sensational ones here. Green tea is potent energizer that contains many, many life-enhancing compounds. It has proven to be anti-cancer, anti-aging, help weight loss and improve vision. It energizes, while relaxing due to

Theanine, an amino acid that actually increases alpha waves in the brain. I prefer to use it instead of black tea because the curing process of black tea destroys many of the Green Tea's life-enhancing qualities. Also Green Tea's stimulating effects are much more long-lasting. I suspect that, like other herbs in this book, further research on Green Tea will continue to wow us all over the years. **Dosage is one or two teabags or one 500 mg capsule extract.**

Reishi:

Reishi mushroom is a powerful immune enhancing herb that has been used in China for untold centuries. Traditionally, like Arjuna, it was used as a heart tonic. It tones the circulatory system and increases Chi (life force) in the face. Like all herbs you want to get them in an organic form if they are available and your bank account permits. It has lately become easy to get this wonderful mushroom in excellent organic form. This herb is not really an energizing herb per se, but will help harmonize the other herbal energizers and have a healthful affect of increasing circulation in the heart center of the body. Most people will notice a soothing and calming effect from this special mushroom with a few hours. **Dosage is 1 or 2 500 mg capsules or 1 500 mg extract capsule.**

Red Dates:
Red Dates or Jujube is a common herb used in Chinese medicine. They have mild sedative qualities but most people won't notice the sedative effect when they use them throughout the day. Red dates are mostly used for their dispersing qualities and can be used with all herbs to help them be more available and useful throughout the body. They are cooling and nurturing to the body. The effects are similar to sweet dates found in the supermarket but Red Dates are more powerful for cooling and dispersing energies. They open the energy pathways in the body so your life-force (Qi) can flow. If your life-force is flowing you are going to have more energy and be healthier. If you buy these in Chinatown look for Red Dates that are thoroughly dried and are free of mold. You can get these in Chinatowns around the country but the easiest way for you may be too to buy wild Jujubi extracts online. Look for an extract that also includes extract from the seeds as this is a very important part of the herb. **Dosage is one 500 mg extract capsule or six dates.**

Rhodiola:

Rhodiola is an herb most people have heard of lately and its effects can be felt by almost anyone in a very short period of time, often within hours of taking it. Most people find it is a great substitute for coffee. Unlike coffee it will not leave you with a feeling of exhaustion at the end of the day and will build a deep sustaining energy in your body overtime. It's so energizing, in fact that I recommend that you don't mix it with coffee, and don't take it in the afternoon. If you do, you may be up all night. If used correctly this herb not only increases energy and vitality throughout the system, but has great health-enhancing and disease preventing qualities. Yes, it is very stimulating, but its most dramatic effects are beyond the stimulation and are felt over time. Try using it for a few weeks to really feel what the herb has to offer. Give it a chance and you'll be happy you did. I think you should always use this herb in extract form to feel its full benefits. Look for an extract that also includes some whole herb. Most people have found that starting at the lowest beginning dosage is a good idea because it is so stimulating. **Dosage is a 250 -500 mg extract capsule.**

Schizandra:

Also known as Wu Wei Tza (pronounced woo way zah) in Chinese. Schizandra has been used in Chinese Medicine for thousands of years. It is a powerful tonic for the whole body. Being of the 'five tastes' it invigorates the entire system. It is said to give healthy glow and brightness to the skin and I believe that it's true. This is one of my favorite herbs and I've have used it successfully for decades. It is not as easy to get quality Schizandra as it is with many other herbs. The best way to obtain Schizandra is to buy it yourself in a Chinatown near you and make a tea. Good quality Schizandra is a deep red color with a slight sheen. If going to Chinatown seems completely impossible to you, some satisfactory extracts are available individually or combined with other complementary herbs. If you do buy Red Dates in Chinatown, a great tea mix would be a rounded teaspoon of the following herbs; Schizandra, Wolfberry and five Red Dates brewed for two hours with 3 cups of water on low heat(just below a simmer). You could also add a small amount of Dendrobium if you wanted. Also, with these whole herb teas you can save and reuse the herbs two more times. It also makes a fine tea as a single herb.

I believe it is an amazing adaptogen and that is even more adaptogenic than Siberian Ginseng! **Dosage is one or two 500 mg capsules or one 500 mg extract tablet or capsule.**

Siberian Ginseng:
Also called Eleuthero or Siberian Eleuthero. Many people taking this don't know it is not really ginseng, in fact, it is not related at all. The effects are not stimulating like regular ginseng but instead work by toning the system and helping it more quickly bounce back from the effects of stress. I personally prefer it over Chinese or Japanese Ginseng because if feels smoother and more compatible with my system. Siberian Ginseng is another herb that has enjoyed a long history of use in China. In China it has traditionally been used to help people move into a healthier sleep pattern over time, (although it is not a sedative), help heart conditions and ease nervous breakdowns. I recommend that you don't use coffee with this herb as it might make you feel over-wired. Of course some people, I've found, like to feel over-wired. **Dosage is one or two 500 mg capsules or 1 500 mg extract capsule.**

Wolfberry:
Wolfberries are also called Goji berries. Wolfberries have really taken off lately as a superfood. Most people know that it if full of antioxidants but that is the extent of their knowledge of this amazing berry. Wolfberries are another herb that has been used in China for thousands of years and is most often paired with Schizandra by herbalists. When used with Schizandra its effects are greatly increased and multiplied. Another thing most people in the west don't know is that it's best when cooked to get the most out of it. By cooking, I mean making a tea from it. If you just chew it you're really missing a lot of it's best effects found in the tiny seeds. The properties in the tiny seed really must be extracted with heat or alcohol extraction. In China it's consumed by millions of people in their daily hot cereal for its longevity and vitality enhancing powers. You may also want to add it to your morning hot cereal to get more out of it. **Dosage is 1 heaping teaspoon in very hot water, adding them to your hot cereal or chewing a rounded teaspoon slowly and thoroughly for up to 5 minutes.**

Turmeric :
Turmeric and curcumin, (a variety of active compounds found in Turmeric) have been

getting an enormous amount of attention lately for their amazing anticancer effects. It has proven to be impossible to give cancer to rats on a high curcumin diet. Most people don't know about its amazing effects on skin and in toning the liver and body. It increases energy overtime so don't expect a dramatic energy enhancing effect immediately. Its energy increasing effects are via its normalizing and harmonizing effect on the entire body and increasing vitality and health throughout the system. I like to take 1 capsule of the whole herb and 1 capsule of extract. **Dosage is one or two 500 mg capsules or one or two 500 mg extract capsule.**

Yarrow:
Yarrow flower is a detoxifier and blood cleaner. It helps to clean impurities out of the system. Over time it helps smooth and de-age the skin. Some people use it as a daily tea but you can get almost all the benefits by taking the powder in capsules. Of course if you are already taking several herbs in powdered form you need to take it as tea because too many capsules of powdered herbs will 'clump' together and probably not be absorbed by the body. I don't think it's necessary to take this herb longer than a few weeks to cleanse and detoxify the body. A good way of taking this

herb is to use it for 3 weeks about 5 times a year. It's easy to get it in excellent powdered form in capsules. One of the most affordable and powerful herbs you can buy!

Dosage is one or two 500 mg capsules or as tea up to 3 times a day.

Chapter 2 Chinese Medicine Simplified

It helps when using herbs to know a little about Chinese medicine. Although many of the herbs mentioned are not always considered Chinese herbs, the following terms can be useful. Remember this is a very simplified explanation of a few Chinese medicinal terms so if this is of interest to you there are many great books available on the subject to expand your knowledge. Even though herbs can have a major impact on restoring energy its wise to be sensitive with the energy you are restoring or depleting. Listen to your body and how you are feeling.

- **Qi:** Qi (pronounced chi) can be described as life force. Qi is the animating force that keeps the organism alive. According to Chinese medicine many illnesses are caused by either a deficiency of Qi or a blockage of Qi. Many herbs increase chi in the body or breakup blockages so that the life force can flow freely. An example would be that Ginger is an herb that helps to breakup blockages and Chinese Ginseng is an herb that increases Qi. Although overtime, an herb could help to disperse blockages sometimes another treatment method is needed such as acupressure or acupuncture.

- **Jing** : Jing is a highly condensed from of essential energy that resides in the kidneys. The amount of Jing in the kidneys throughout one's life is said to determine one's lifespan and play a major role in the health of the individual. Activities that can lead to loss of Jing include working too hard for an extended period of time, overindulgence in any activity that severely exhausts you especially when combined with lack of sleep and constantly forcing your body to go beyond its limits. Even too much exercise, like too many races for a runner could lead to a loss of Jing. A person may be born with more Jing, so they would be able to handle more stress over time. Some herbs that help restore Jing are Dendrobium, Gokshura, Schizandra , Cordyceps and He Sho Wu. Some forms of Qigong (a Chinese moving mediation), deep breathing and deep sleep can also contribute to restoring Jing.

- **Yin and Yang:** Yin can be seen as cooling while Yang could be seen as heating. A healthy individual needs to have a balance of yin and yang energy circulating through their system to stay healthy. While many herbs can have a neutral energy, many have warming (yang) or cooling (yin) properties. Ginger and Cinnamon could be seen as a hot (yang) while Red Dates and Wolfberries could be seen as a Yin herb. Yang is also associated with fire properties and the heart and Yin is associated with water properties and the kidneys. Many herbs have properties of both. Which energy predominates would depend on how it is prepared or which herbs are combined.
- **Energy Meridians:** Energy meridians are focal points in the body where bodily energies accumulate and concentrate. They could also be called chakras. These can't be seen or studied with medical instruments but they definitely are real and important. Blockages and or deficiencies of energy in the meridians can cause low energy and accelerated aging. Energy channels in the body concentrate in the

meridians. Herbs as well as certain exercises, such as qigong, clear and enhance the functioning of these meridians.

- **Energy Channels**: Energy channels run throughout the body carrying life force (Qi) through our systems. They connect at points called acupuncture points or tsubos. If these meeting points get blocked we can get sick or just not feel great. Sometimes a person has tons of natural energy, but a point or points that are sluggish or blocked will cause them to feel tired. When the points along the energy channels are flowing and abundant a person will feel healthy and free of pain. Some of the ways of unblocking them include certain types of yoga, massage, qigong, acupressure and acupuncture. Simply rubbing a point, if you know where it is, can also help.

Chapter 3 How to Use the Herbs

The best way to take the herbs is to take them regularly and in significant amounts. You can't take them every other day and expect to have as powerful effect as taking them everyday. You will have some effect, but I don't think you will be satisfied with it.

Often, over the years, many people have asked me for recommendations on which herbs to take, knowing my reputation and level of vitality. Most people will take the herbs for a few days, or over a couple of weeks on the outside and then stop. They assume they will work like magical drugs and have an instant and miraculous effect like a super drug. Some herbs do have very dramatic and instant effects and some take time to reveal their inner magic. When many people don't see an obvious and dramatic effect they quit. Eventually they end up throwing them out when they clean their cupboards out. Some herbs really can have an immediate and dramatic effect (especially some of the extracts) and you feel and see the results in a few hours or days, but the majority takes time to harmonize with your system and slowly produces obvious results. Those that are patient and give them at least 30 days will be extremely happy with the result. I say give them 3 months and then decide. It's worth the wait. But don't see it as waiting; see it as investing in a powerful and vitality filled new you.

The extracts referred to in this book are a powerfully intense form and I think you should really only use them once a day, preferably in the morning upon a waking, with a full glass of water. These herbs are highly concentrated and may actually have the opposite effect intended if you use them more than once a day. Taking the extracts once a day is really all you need especially if you are taking more than one, as combining them greatly enhances the effects of each.

Don't try to use too many herbs at the same time when beginning. Start with 3 or 4 herbs and see how that works for you. You could even start with one of the most powerful herbs such as Ashwagandha or Rhodiola and see if you are even interested in using herbs. It might actually be a major advantage to start with one of these herbs in extract form so you can see more a dramatic and undeniable effect. Pay attention to how you feel. If you are feeling to warm throughout the day back off on some of the warming herbs. If you are feeling to cool throughout the day you can increase the warming herbs. My recommendation is to begin a practice of stopping what you are doing a couple times a day and pay attention to what your feeling. Your body is intuitive and smart it will communicate its status to you if you are listening. **Remember not all herbs feel or work the same way for everybody, so don't expect them too!** I think this is one of the failings of the western medicine model. Everyone really is unique and responds to natural or western medicine practices in the own way. Investigate your uniqueness! Below are some herbal combinations that work for many.

Powder or Extract

I like to use extracts for their quick acting effects. A powder takes longer to get into your system, as your body has to do its own extraction process over a period of time. The whole process of getting into your system could actually take between 1 to 3 hours. Much longer if you take it with food. A quality extract capsule will begin to open in less and 30 seconds and in a very short period of time the extract begins to be absorbed by the intestinal tract. I do take powdered herbs everyday though, but use extracts when I want a quick and reliable potency released in my system.

Also if you take too many capsules of powdered herb at the same time they could form a thick pasty mix that could move very slowly through your system and may not be well absorbed at all. Of course if you take extract alone you might be missing some of the herbal cofactors that naturally occur to improve the herbs effects in the human system. It is very likely that as the herbs are studied in the future amazing compounds will be found that are not found in current extracts. So what to take? I think that the best choice is to take both whenever possible. Take an extract that includes whole herbs or purchase the powdered form and extract and take them at the same time. Another thing you can do is make your own extracts of the herbs by putting a slightly rounded teaspoon of the herb (not ginger as it is too strong) in the bottom of a tea cup, add 8 oz of very hot water (not boiling), cover and drink it when it cools. Fresh extract is usually the best way to go if you have the time. You could also alternate your fresh tea extract with a commercial extract if you're a really busy person.

Organic or Non-organic

Only recently has organic been an option for medicinal herbs. In the past people just bought herbs and were happy at their availably. Now when many consumers think of buying natural products like herbs, they think about organic first. I always choose organic produce when I can get it and it looks fresh, but this is not my first choice when it comes to purchasing herbs. Organic produce has been available for decades and they have perfected and streamlined the process. In most places its easy and reasonable to choose organic produce, but I personally don't think this is currently an important consideration when choosing herbs. For one thing the availably of organic herbs is extremely limited. Only a few of the major herbs like Turmeric and garlic and few others can be found in organic form. Also it's important to know that many of the herbs you'll be using in this book are cultivated using methods that are hundreds of years old. Most herbs on the market today are the product of generations of pride in choosing and producing the best quality herbs a family or village can produce. They are usually cultivated using the best resources and methods that are available to them and the result is typically superior in quality. I have found that some of the newer organic herbs are often inferior in quality and potency because herb growers are forced to use methods that are unfamiliar to them to get the organic certification.

Currently I think the best way to get a good quality herb is to buy from a reputable manufacturer that I have listed in the back of book.

Some Useful combinations

- Schizandra, Siberian Ginseng and Wolfberry
- Ashwagandha, Siberian Ginseng and Green Tea
- Schizandra, Wolfberries and Ginger (for cold constitutions)
- Wolfberries and Red Dates (for hot constitutions)
- Reishi, Wolfberries and Green Tea
- Schizandra, Wolfberries and Red Dates
- Ginger and Green Tea
- Cordyceps and Green Tea
- Rhodiola and Siberian Ginseng

- Wolfberries, Red Dates and Dendrobium (for cooling, restoration and longevity)
- Ginger and Cayenne (for cold constitutions)
- Cinnamon and Ginger (for cold constitutions)
- Wolfberries, Red Dates and American Ginseng (for hot constitutions)

I didn't include Turmeric in these combinations because it really is just something you should always take every day.

Chapter 4 Ways to Get the Most from Your Herbs

I've included this small chapter to help people get the most out of their herbs. It's short and sweet, but important.

- Take the herbs everyday.
- Start with one herb for at least 2 weeks before deciding whether you want to keep taking it.
- Take at least a full 8 oz glass of water when taking the herbs or they may ball up in a gluey mess that just doesn't get absorbed. Don't take a sip of water with the herbs (as my best friend often does) and expect to get much benefit.
- If you are taking more than 2 capsules of powdered herb (extracts are okay) at one time take them on an empty stomach as they may not open at all or open so far down in your digestive track where they aren't going to do you any good and might make you feel sick.
- It's a good idea not to take stimulating herbs like Rhodiola or

Green Tea extracts late in the day unless you want to be up late. I know this is true because once I didn't want to miss a day on my herb regimen and took both of these late, and I was up all night.

- Consider taking a course or adopting an activity that stretches the energy channels and opens energy meridians in the body. Allowing the herbs energies to circulate through the system and be utilized properly. Some of the best activities would be qigong, yoga, brisk walking and running.

- Look to establish your current constitution. Do you get cold often when everyone around you feels fine? If so you might have a cold or Yin nature and may benefit more by using herbal combinations that warm you. Do you feel hot often when most people feel fine? Then it's possible that you have a warm or hot constitution and could benefit the most from the Yin or cooling herbs. Because everyone is unique this is something best decided by you with the possible help of a qualified acupuncturist or herbalist with a Chinese herb background.

Chapter 5 Buy Good Quality Herbs

You usually get what you pay for so pay a little more for good brands. It will cost more but it will mean the difference between herbs that work and herbs that don't. I never buy my herbs supplements at the grocery store, pharmacy or a liquor store. These places just don't usually carry good herbs and if you do find good quality herbs at these stores the prices are usually full retail. I love to buy my Chinese herbs in a local Chinatown or Asian market. I love the smell of these markets and the whole wonderful atmosphere but I know that the average person would be lost in these environments and wouldn't be able to recognize low quality from high quality. If you do want to explore this way of buying the Chinese herbs, price usually determines quality. As a rule the highest price means highest quality and lowest price means lowest quality. For most people buying online is the best way to go initially. Buy online and you can get your herbs at nearly half the price or more! Some of the most popular and high quality brands and companies I use are listed below. They are considered some of the most reliable herb producing companies around and have great reputations.

Nature's Way (for herbs and herbal extracts)

Now Foods (herbs and herb extracts)

Gaia (for herbal extracts)

Planetary Formulas (herbal extracts often mixed with whole herbs)

Questions and Answers

These are a few of the more common questions I get asked about herbs.

Question: When is the best time to take the herbs?

I found that the best time to take the herbs is in the morning with your morning beverage, especially if you have a busy schedule. The herbs can also be taken a second or third time in the day, to have a faster effect, but I have found that most people will quit taking the herbs if they have to follow a regimen like this. Its better to make the herbs in one convenient daily dose than have a person abandon their herbs. It may take longer to feel the effects of some of the slower acting herbs, but I think you'll be happier this way in the long run because you're more likely to continue your herb program.

Question: How many herbs can I take at one time?

You can take several herbs at once but I recommend that you only take a few herbs to start or even one so you don't feel overwhelmed or get tired of the schedule. Make it easy on yourself and start out slow. As I stated in an earlier chapter you might want to start with one of the powerful herbs such as Aswaganda or Rhodiloa in extract form to really feel the power of herbs so you will know that herbs are extremely useful and potent.

Question: Are herbs expensive?

The answer is it depends on what you choose to take. The more herbs you take the more you spend. Also some of the herbs take longer to cultivate and process which results in a higher cost. In addition, the powdered and powdered capsuled herbs cost a lot less than the extracts. This makes sense because it takes 10 times or of the powdered herb to make one capsule of extract. I don't feel herbs are that expensive at all considering their long term affect on energy, vitality and the most important effect of longevity. Keep in mind that you really don't need to take all the herbs listed in this book to have a dramatic affect on your life.

Question: I don't feel anything. When will I notice something?

I think this is the most common question I get and I usually get it a couple of days after a person starts taking the herbs. I have to say, and your probably expecting this, it really does depend on the person. These are powerful substances and you will notice an effect pretty quickly if you are just a little patient. Your not drinking espresso (although some people think Rhodiola extract offers a similar rush) so try not to expect it to feel that rush. Most of these are classed as tonic herbs and that means they help to put your body into a healthier and stronger state when taken over a long period of time. Also, I have to ask how sensitive are you to how your body is changing and gaining benefit? If you are drinking a lot of coffee or energy drinks your body has been pushed past its limits and you may not feel the benefit right away, even if it is very significant. I don't want you to misunderstand me. These herbs are incredible and everyone, I mean everyone, will feel the effects in time if you keep taking the herbs. Herbs are wonderful, be patient and find out for yourself as I have.

Question: How long can I take the herbs?

This is probably not something you really need to think about right now. As you become more familiar with the herbs you'll know what you like and what you don't like. As I've stated earlier these herbs should be taken over a prolonged period of time and some people may wish to take a few for the rest of their life for longevity benefits such as Turmeric , Wolfberry and Schizandra.

Question: How do herbs work?

Herbs work in many ways through naturally occurring chemical-like substances that are products of the original plant. Many of the herb plants contain thousands of these substances that powerfully affect a living body. I also believe that there is so much more to it than just plant chemicals working on us. I feel that the plants have unique energies that influence us in profound ways. It's clear to me that these energies are carried through our body's energy channels and meridians, doing their magic, while on the surface it appears like it's just a matter of interesting plant chemicals interacting with us. I'm sure this will be more thoroughly investigated by science in the not too distant future. The more you work and understand the herbs the more it becomes easier to believe that they were actually intelligently designed to be used by humans for medicine and dynamic health.

Question: How do I make a tea from dry herbs?

If the herb is in powdered form and you want to get it in your system quickly, open a capsule of the powdered herb, or put a teaspoon of the powder in the bottom of a teacup and add 8 ounces of very hot water and let it steep for 5 minutes before sipping.

If the herb is in dry whole form that is non-ground, take a heaping teaspoon of one or more herbs and add them to 3 cups of water and cook (water should be just below simmering) covered in a high quality glass* pot for 2 to 3 hours. Try to drink this brew within 2 days to maintain potency. This a traditional practice and possibly the best way to extract the properties from the herbs.

Question: Can herbs heal me?
The simple answer is yes when used by someone who knows what herb to use and when and how to apply it. I've seen and heard about shamans doing incredible healings with herbs. It's good to remember

though, that all healing is self healing and that by healing, I mean the herb or herbs were used in a way to remove or eliminate energy blocks in a body so that the body can quickly restore itself. Also some herbs such as Garlic and Olive Leaf are fantastic antibiotics that kill pathogens invading the system. TCM or traditional Chinese medicine is all about using herbs for healing when combined with acupuncture. The real focus of this book is about making yourself healthier, increasing your longevity and increasing your personal strength and power.

*It is recommended that you don't use a metal pot as this can possibly affect the potency of the herbal brew.

Herbal Resources

This section covers online sites that sell vitamins and supplements. I have no financial interest in any of these companies. I have found these to be the cheapest and most convenient places for me to buy the herbs used in this book. Most are known for shipping fast and offer discounts on shipping, especially if you order a large amount at one time. I switch between these companies if one doesn't have what I want in stock.

- **Amazon.com** They offer a wide variety of supplements and almost always carry the herbs described in this book. Just make sure it is actually being sold by Amazon when you order as they also allow other companies to sell through their website. Other companies, I have found, may not be as reliable as Amazon.
- **Vitacost** I use this company often and they have a reputation for reliability. Reviews show a high customer satisfaction.
- **iHerb** This is another company I use often when I can't find the

products I need from the above companies.

- **Swanson Vitamins** Another company that sometimes has the best prices. One issue that sometimes comes up is that if your order is less than a pound it may be shipped very slowly with no tracking available. Also it is always advisable to pay the extra shipping charge of a few dollars when ordering, to get your products in a timely manner.

- **Chinese Herbs Direct** I often buys herbs and herbal combinations from this online company when I can't get to a Chinatown. They ship quickly, have good prices and even carry some American herbs and American herbal formulas.

- **Wing Hop Fung** When I used to frequent the herbs stores in the Los Angeles Chinatown this was always one of my favorite places to go. They are very friendly to American visitors and are patient when you try to correctly pronounce the herbs in Chinese. Also, their prices are very fair. They have a wide selection of wonderful Green Teas upstairs. However, I have never used their online shop so I can't vouch for how well it functions.

Conclusion

Herbs do wonderful things in the body when used in significant amounts over time. I've seen incredible changes in people that embrace the herbs and use them properly. A person can transform their physical well being and energy in just a few months of daily use. When you are patient long enough to see and feel the real power of these herbs, you'll keep using them for life.

Healthy Journeys

About The Author

Richard Anderson has done extensive research into alternative healing practices. As a child he suffered from several near fatal illnesses that left him with a sense of urgency in exploring alternative methods of healing and staying well. He has spent decades exploring many forms of alternative healing, including Ayurvedic medicine, herbal medicine, Traditional Chinese medicine, acupressure, reflexology, nutritional healing and vitamin therapy. He is also proficient in Quantum Touch and is a Reiki master. He is continually searching cutting edge breakthroughs in alternative healing. He believes it's best to use a combination of healing modalities to bring the body back to harmony.

www.brightpath.org